Get Rid Of Low Back Pain

TABLE OF CONTENTS

What You Can Expect 7

Back in Balance 9

Before You Begin 10

Secrets of Your Back
The Spine & The Vertebrae 12

The Best Way to Treat Your Back 17

Say Goodbye to Your Low Back Pain 22

A Word of Caution 28

Well Done!!! 29

Get Rid Of Low Back Pain

Get Rid Of Low Back Pain

This resource has been provided to you by **Superior Rehabilitation**. We would like to be your choice for all your physical therapy needs. Our staff takes great pride in treating your symptoms with the latest technology that is available while staying current with new trends. We treat patients of all ages from children to adults with an expertise in orthopedics. Based on your specific needs, your treatment may include: therapeutic exercises, unweighted ambulation, manual therapy, soft tissue manipulation including myofascial release, Graston Technique, Trigger Point Dry Needling, Kinesiotape, athletic taping, neuromuscular and interferential electrical stimulation, iontophoresis, ultrasound and more. We also address issues with balance impairments.

Contact our clinic at 504-887-7463 for a **FREE Consultation** to see if physical therapy can help you restore your body's function.

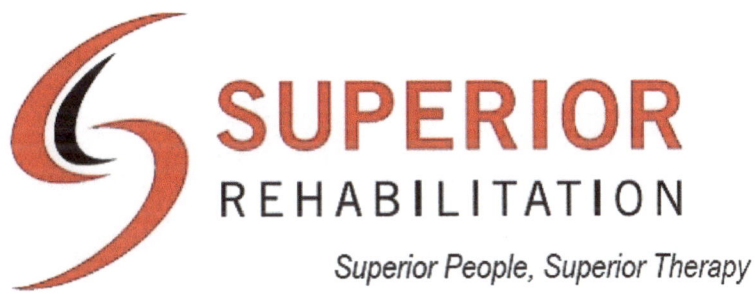

MIKE MCNEIL, PT, DPT, ATC

6820 VETERANS BLVD. STE. A

METAIRIE, LA 70003

CLINIC (504) 887-7463

FAX (504) 887-7115

Disclaimer

The information in this book is not a replacement for the services of a physician or health care professional.

Please do not use this book to diagnose or treat a medical or health condition.

Please consult a physician in all matters relating to your health, and use discretion when using any of the strategies mentioned here.

Dear Patient,

Thank you for choosing to read this book. I have compiled this as a quick resource to enable you to deal with low back pain. Statistics show that a large number of adults exhibit back pain symptoms every year. The severity of low back pain can range from mild to severe, and can, in some cases, cause symptoms of nerve compression (lack of sensation or paralysis) if left untreated.

In addition to finding useful information on lower back pain in this book, you will be pleased to learn that you are now on our exclusive newsletter subscriber list.

This entitles you to some cutting edge information on health, wellness and injury prevention, all delivered to you at regular intervals.

Get Rid Of Low Back Pain

Each edition will feature valuable tips, health plans, expert advice and informative articles to keep you healthy and live without pain. You can share this excellent resource of healthy living with your acquaintances, by forwarding it to their email address or asking them to sign up, FREE for them. This newsletter is our commitment to improving your health as your preferred healthcare professional.

Thank you!

WHAT YOU CAN EXPECT

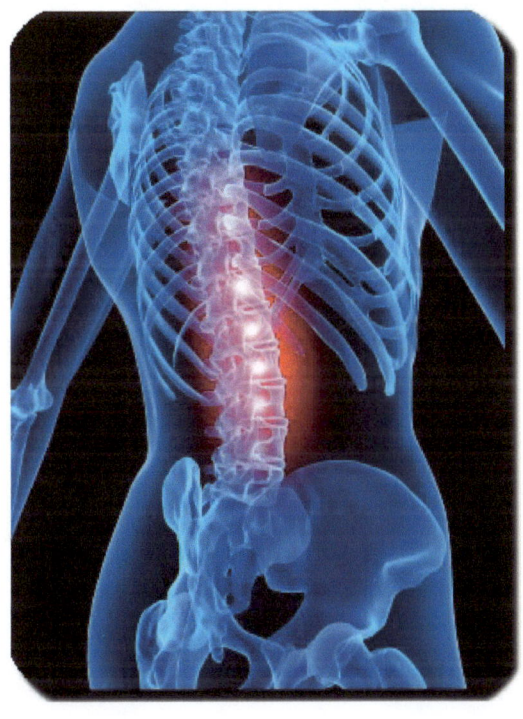

The goal of this book is to help you maintain the right spinal alignment on a daily basis. Over a period of time, you will notice that your posture improves and you will experience an increased sense of comfort while driving and performing day to day activities. Within a few weeks, you will find yourself adjusting your posture for all activities, including work, travel and household chores to maximize the comfort and minimize the strain on the lower back.

The exercises you are about to learn will help you develop self-awareness and improved posture. Since all physical activities require your spine to be in its optimum shape, these exercises serve several purposes and build a foundation for long term strength and well being.

With regular exercise, the flexibility of your lower back will improve. You may experience some discomfort; however, this is a normal consequence of properly executed exercises. Over a period of time, discomfort will reduce. This implies your lower back is getting stronger and becoming more functional.

BACK IN BALANCE

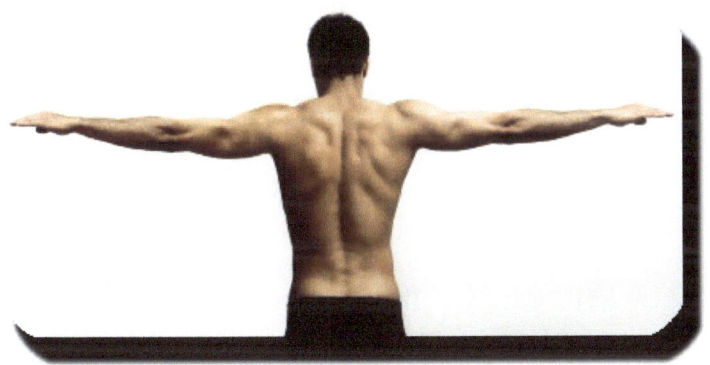

The above picture reflects a straight back with properly developed and balanced muscles around the spine. This facilitates optimum balance and posture in the lower back. It is important to exercise muscles evenly on all sides to develop and maintain **muscle balance**. In addition, the blood circulation around the vertebrae and the inter-vertebral discs will also improve. As a result, the lower back becomes stronger and more flexible!

BEFORE YOU BEGIN

Always consult a physician or a licensed healthcare professional, like a physical therapist, before starting an exercise plan to determine if you are ready to start exercising.

All the exercises mentioned in this book are designed to relieve pain in your lower back. Therefore, if an exercise is increasing the pain, please discontinue and consult a certified provider.

Caution: If you experience pain during an exercise, discontinue it. Proceed with the other exercises in the routine. A few days later, try the same exercise again. If it is still painful, drop it from your routine for some time.

In the early stages, you may not be able to repeat an exercise to the specified count, but do not allow that to discourage you. As the lower back gets stronger and more flexible, you will reach the right strength level.

Let us start by learning more about the structure of the spine. This will help understand the lower back and its movements in greater detail.

SECRETS OF YOUR BACK, THE SPINE & THE VERTEBRAE

The spine provides the structural framework to the entire body. The spinal cord runs through the middle of the spine and serves as the main highway of the nervous system by connecting the brain with other parts of the body. The vertebrae of the spine surround and protect the spinal cord.

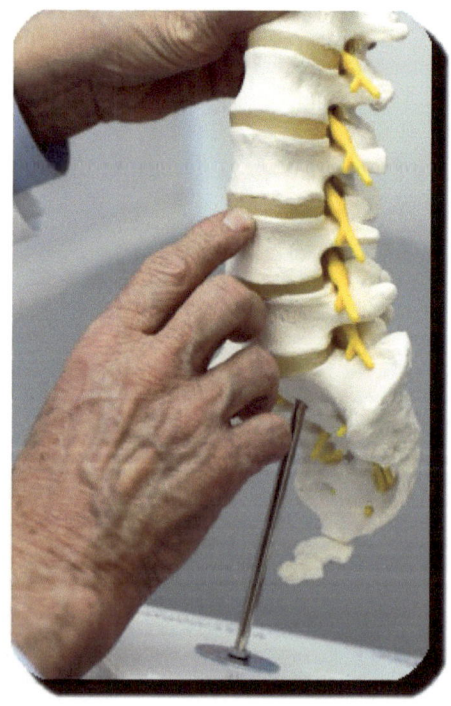

It is imperative to keep the spine healthy and in good shape. When seen from the side, a normal spine reveals an S-shape. This unique curvature effectively absorbs forces of varying nature and intensity that are exerted on the body in an average day.

Similar to shock absorbers in a car, the spine transforms shocks into movement. This movement of the spine, in case of an external impact, is facilitated by its S-shaped curvature. If the spine were completely straight, the impact would affect the vertebral discs directly. As a result, the vertebral discs would wear out much sooner and expose the spinal cord to the peril of these forces.

Therefore, a healthy back is similar to a shock absorption system that transforms force into movement within the reach of the S-shape.

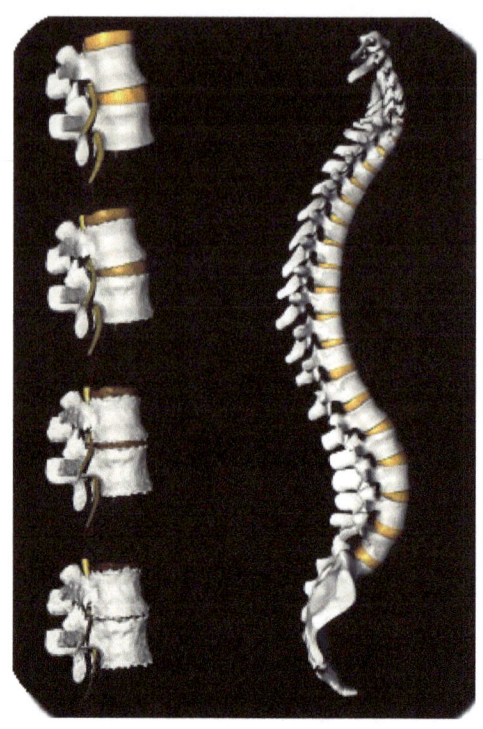

A stiff lower back does not move easily and causes too much exertion on the vertebral discs leading to excessive disc compression. When your lower back is accustomed to the wrong posture (neglect), it cannot absorb shock without causing damage to the discs.

The vertebrae of the back are not simply stacked on top of each other but are separated by small elastic discs, similar to tiny cushions.

Healthy discs are elastic, a little "squishy," and make up 20-25% of the total length of the vertebral column. A vertebral disc is made of a gel-like center (nucleus pulposi) and an outer wall (annulus fibrosus). Healthy vertebral discs consist of almost 90% water, just as in healthy infants. As one grows older, the body is unable to retain optimum water level in the discs. In a stiff lower back, the vertebral discs are more susceptible to drying out and become thinner. To maintain optimum hydration of the vertebral discs, good blood circulation in the vertebral region is necessary. **This is achieved by a sustained and progressive use of the muscles surrounding the vertebrae.**

A lower back without sufficient movement does not get enough blood circulation and causes insufficient hydration of the discs. Discs in a rigid lower back, therefore, thin out faster as there is no shock absorption mechanism in place to stop them from wearing out.

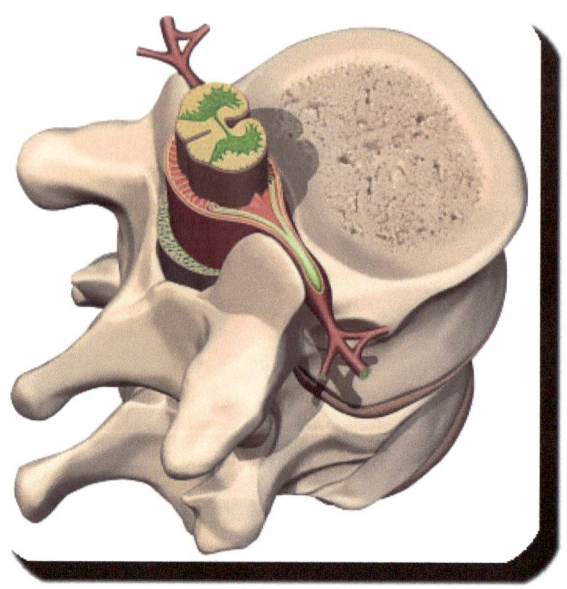

Remember: good circulation = good hydration.

Without adequate movement and exercise, people tend to become overweight, which places additional strain on the discs and reduces blood supply to them. Thinner discs tend to slip out of position in the vertebrae easily and weak muscles are completely ineffective to prevent this from happening.

The Best Way To Treat Your Back

Research shows that the best way to treat the lower back is by increasing mobility and strength in a progressive, controlled manner.

This requires a plan to:

1) Strengthen muscles, so they can bring and keep vertebrae in position and

2) Increase blood circulation around the discs, thereby allowing the discs to suck up all the fluid they need to make the lower back supple.

For best results, an exercise program should stress:

1. Increasing mobility of the back
2. Aligning the vertebrae
3. Increasing circulation
4. Decompression of the discs
5. Strengthening of the muscles

The exercises in this book are in line with the above goals.

A sedentary lifestyle is one of the main reasons for low back pain. Lack of physical exercise, poor posture and excessive sitting are only a few of the many factors that strain the lower back. Lower back pain is an early symptom of future back problems like a herniated disc or a frozen back.

Fortunately, a well planned routine of exercises for the lower back can assist in restoring the spine or getting it closer to its original, painless and functional state. The secret to regaining a normal, functional spine is training the muscles of the lower back and strengthening them to keep a healthy posture. Strong and supple muscles will keep the lower back in good shape for a long time.

It is important for your body to maintain the right posture at all times. The muscles of the body have to be trained to achieve the natural posture for sitting and working. The following are the guidelines that help train muscles to keep a healthy posture while sitting.

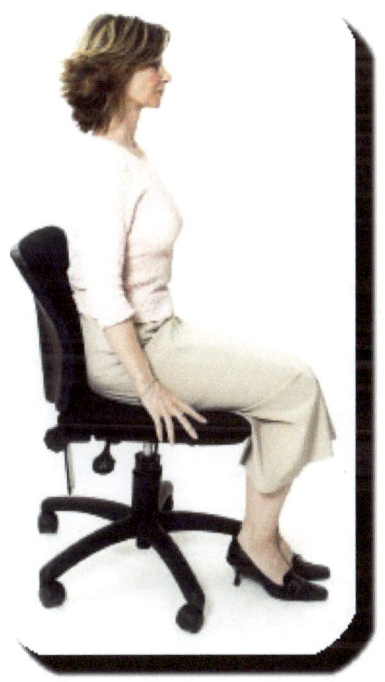

- Lower arm should extend horizontally

- The knee-hollow should not touch the edge of the chair

- Lower back should be sufficiently supported

- A display should be on a natural height at eye level

- Elbows should be supported by the armrests of the chair

- Feet should lie flat on the ground

If you suffer from a bulging or herniated disc, here are some areas that your healthcare professional will help you focus on: (1) mobilize the back, (2) align the back, (3) decompress the spine, (4) strengthen the muscle of the back, and (5) maintain a healthy diet.

Clearly, four out of the five areas require exercising on a regular basis; therefore, exercise is the first and most important step in treating lower back problems.

People suffering from a herniated disc should start exercising in a very controlled manner. It is advisable to start under the vigilance of a physician or an exercise professional like a physical therapist.

Say Goodbye to Your Low Back Pain

Here are some recommendations for a core strengthening exercise routine. Always consult your physical therapist to get a customized exercise program best suited for your specific needs.

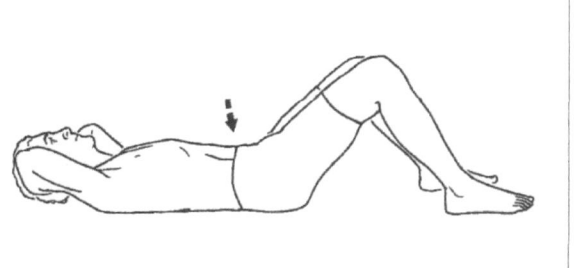

PELVIC TILT

Lying down on your back, bend your knees to where your feet are flat on the floor or mat. Flatten your back by tightening the muscles of your stomach and buttocks. Hold 2-3 seconds. Repeat 10 times per set and do 3 sets.

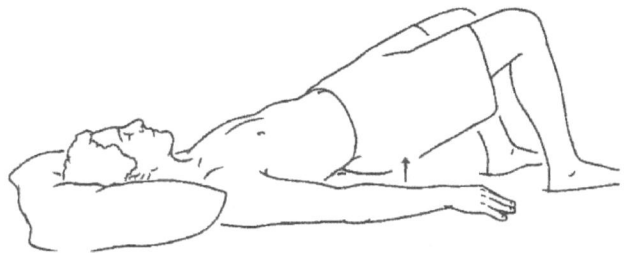

BRIDGING

In this same position, hold your arms on the ground next to your body and slowly raise your buttocks from the floor, keeping your stomach muscles tight. Go up until you feel your tailbone and one vertebra at a time come off the ground. When only the back of your shoulders are touching the ground, maintain this position (with abdominals tight) for 2-3 seconds and then relax. Repeat this exercise 10 times per set and do 3 sets.

Get Rid Of Low Back Pain

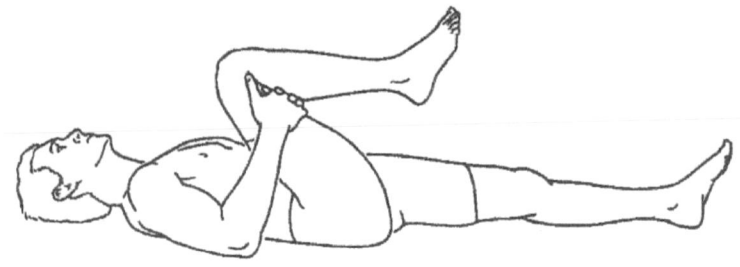

KNEE-TO-CHEST STRETCH

Lie down flat on the floor with your left foot resting flat against it and your right leg straight. With your hand behind the left knee, pull knee slowly into your chest until a comfortable stretch is felt in the lower back and buttocks. Keep your back relaxed. Hold 10 seconds. Repeat the same process 10 times, and then perform with your other leg 10 times.

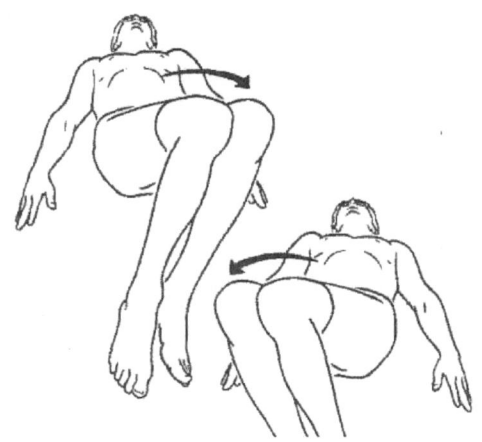

LOWER TRUNK ROTATION

Lie down flat on the floor with your feet resting flat on the ground and your knees bent. Slowly rock your knees from side to side in small, pain-free range of motion. Allow lower back to rotate slightly. Repeat this exercise 10 times per set and do 3 sets.

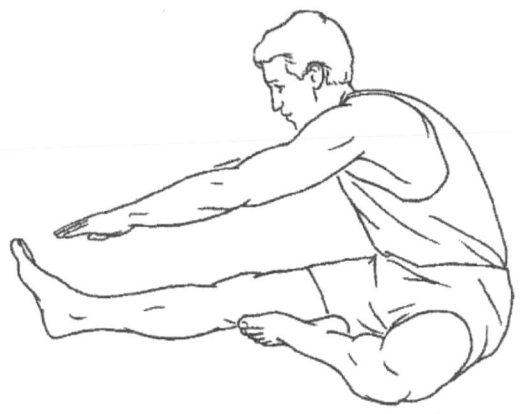

HAMSTRING STRETCH

Start in a seated position with your left leg bent, but keeping your right leg straight. Reach down along right leg until a comfortable stretch is felt in the back of your thigh. Be sure to keep your knee straight. Hold 30 seconds. Switch legs to stretch your left hamstring as well. Repeat this stretch 3 times with each leg.

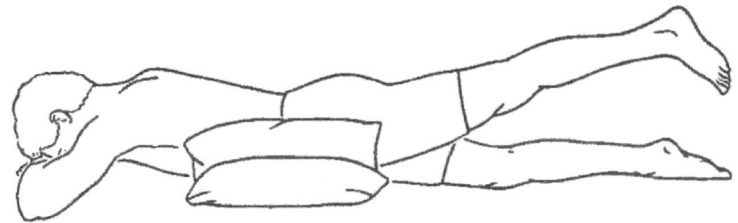

HIP EXTENSION (PRONE)

Lie down flat with your face down and position a pillow under your stomach. Lift your left leg 12 inches from the surface, keeping your knee straight. Repeat with your right leg. Continue with this exercise alternating kicks with each leg, as if you were swimming. Perform 10 times with each leg per set and do 3 sets.

A Word of Caution

The above exercises increase blood circulation around the hips and the lower back. Increased circulation will help heal the discs of the lower back and increase the blood supply to the muscles you are training in this area. Your pelvis and SI-joint also benefit from the increased blood circulation in their region. These exercises may seem very simple, but they work well to restore mobility in the lower back.

If any of these exercises increase pain, or cause tingling or numbness of the limbs or back, stop immediately and consult a licensed physical therapist. In such cases, there will be some modifications made to the exercises specific to your spine's condition. If you have any questions regarding your diagnosis, feel free to ask your physical therapist.

W<u>ELL DONE!!!</u>

Congratulations on taking the right steps to improve the health of your lower back. These were some exercises designed to put you on a track to healthy life by relieving the pain in the lower back.

www.ingramcontent.com/pod-product-compliance
Lightning Source LLC
Chambersburg PA
CBHW041615180526
45159CB00002BC/872